GASTRIC S

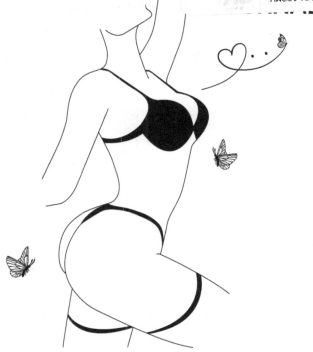

THIS BOOK BELONGS TO:

NAME:

....

....

ADDRESS:

....

....

....

PHONE & EMAIL:

....

....

....

MY MEASUREMENTS

	BEFORE	AFTER		BEFORE	AFTER
WAIST			NECK		
CHEST			HIPS		
THIGH			BUST		
CALF			ARM		

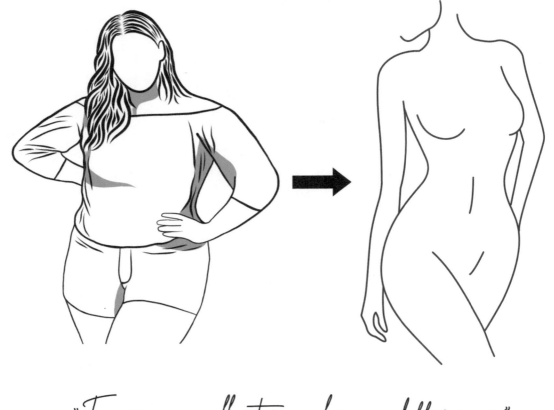

"Every small step makes a difference."

Thank you very much for purchasing this book.
If you find the book helpful, consider **leaving a Review on Amazon.**
Your valuable feedback will help others and encourage us to create more quality products.

MY STARTING PHOTO
Glue in the latest photo of yourself before surgery!
So you can look back at it at the end of your journey to be amazed!

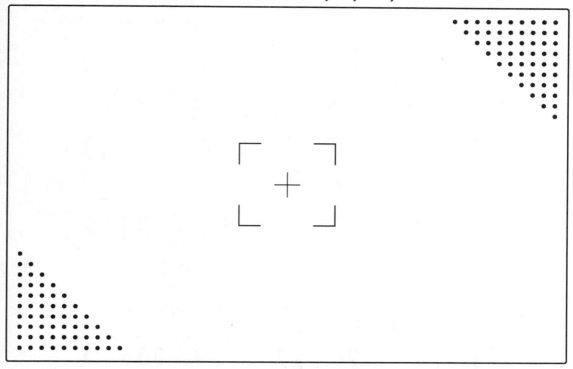

PHOTO OF "THE NEW ME"
Glue in the newest photo of yourself after two months of your journey!
So you can see the amazing result you have done so far!

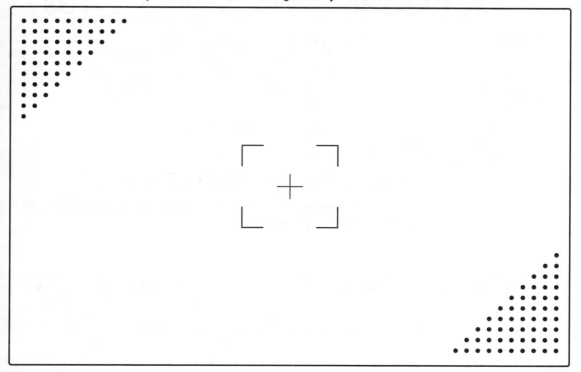

MY FIRST 50 POUND

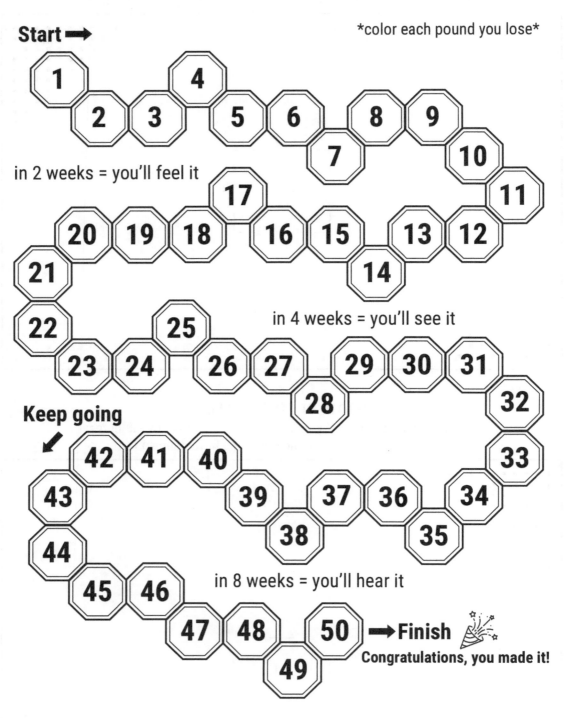

color each pound you lose

Start ➡

Keep going

in 2 weeks = you'll feel it

in 4 weeks = you'll see it

in 8 weeks = you'll hear it

➡ Finish 🎉
Congratulations, you made it!

"You have always been beautiful, since now you are just deciding to be healthier, fitter, faster, and stronger. Remember that"

MY VISION BOARD

HEALTH

SOCIAL

WELLNESS

FUN

SUCCESS

OTHER:

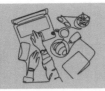

WEEKLY ACTIVITY PLANNER

WEEK OF: ....

WEEKLY CHALLENGES AND GOALS

- ☐ ....
- ☐ ....
- ☐ ....
- ☐ ....
- ☐ ....
- ☐ ....
- ☐ ....
- ☐ ....
- ☐ ....
- ☐ ....
- ☐ ....
- ☐ ....
- ☐ ....
- ☐ ....
- ☐ ....
- ☐ ....
- ☐ ....
- ☐ ....
- ☐ ....
- ☐ ....
- ☐ ....
- ☐ ....

WEEKLY TO-DO LISTS

- ☐ ....
- ☐ ....
- ☐ ....
- ☐ ....
- ☐ ....
- ☐ ....
- ☐ ....
- ☐ ....
- ☐ ....
- ☐ ....
- ☐ ....
- ☐ ....

- ☐ ....
- ☐ ....
- ☐ ....
- ☐ ....
- ☐ ....
- ☐ ....
- ☐ ....
- ☐ ....
- ☐ ....
- ☐ ....
- ☐ ....
- ☐ ....

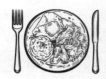

WEEKLY MEAL PLANNER

WEEK OF: ....

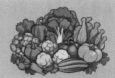

	BREAKFAST	SNACK	LUNCH	DINNER
MON				
TUE				
WED				
THU				
FRI				
SAT				
SUN				

DAILY PROGRESS & TRACKER

Date: ....

Day:........... of my journey   Weight: ....   Mo - Tu - We - Th - Fr - Sa - Su

Daily affirmations: ....
....
....

Today mood: 😊 😄 😎 😐 😳 😵 😖

	Low	Medium	High
Energy level	☐	☐	☐
Sleep quality	☐	☐	☐
Stress level	☐	☐	☐
Activity level	☐	☐	☐

Today's goals:
☐ ....
☐ ....
☐ ....

Medications:
☐ ....
☐ ....
☐ ....

Supplements/Nutrition:
☐ ....
☐ ....
☐ ....

Water intake (1 cup = 8 oz)

Coffee I drank today

Juice I drank today

Meditation: from: .... to: .... total minutes: ....

Cardio: from: .... to: .... total calories burn: ....

Exercise: from: .... to: .... total minutes: ....
Type: ....

Daily events
☐ ....   ☐ ....
☐ ....   ☐ ....
☐ ....   ☐ ....

Daily important notes
....
....
....
....
....
....
....

DAILY FOOD LOG

Food	Amount	Cal	Protein	Carbs	Fats	Sugar
Breakfast time:................						
Lunch time:................						
Dinner time:................						
Snacks time:						

FOOD TRIGGER TRACKER

Immediately after	After 1 hour	After 3 hours

Symptoms/Pains: ....
....
....
....
....
....
....

DAILY PROGRESS & TRACKER

Date: ....

Day: .... of my journey   Weight: ....

Mo - Tu - We - Th - Fr - Sa - Su

Daily affirmations: ....
....
....

	Low	Medium	High
Energy level	☐	☐	☐
Sleep quality	☐	☐	☐
Stress level	☐	☐	☐
Activity level	☐	☐	☐

Today mood: ☺ ☺ 😎 ☺ 😴 🤪 😖

Today's goals:
☐ ....
☐ ....
☐ ....

Medications:
☐ ....
☐ ....
☐ ....

Supplements/Nutrition:
☐ ....
☐ ....
☐ ....

Water intake (1 cup = 8 oz)

Coffee I drank today

Juice I drank today

Meditation: from: .... to: .... total minutes: ....

Cardio: from: .... to: .... total calories burn: ....

Exercise: from: .... to: .... total minutes: ....
Type: ....

Daily events
☐ .... ☐ ....
☐ .... ☐ ....
☐ .... ☐ ....

Daily important notes
....
....
....
....
....
....
....

DAILY FOOD LOG

Food	Amount	Cal	Protein	Carbs	Fats	Sugar
🍳 Breakfast time:.................						
🌐 Lunch time:.................						
🍽 Dinner time:.................						
🍪 Snacks time:						

FOOD TRIGGER TRACKER

Immediately after	After 1 hour	After 3 hours

Symptoms/Pains: ....
....
....
....
....
....
....

DAILY PROGRESS & TRACKER

Date: ....

Day: .... of my journey   Weight: ....   Mo - Tu - We - Th - Fr - Sa - Su

Daily affirmations: ....
....
....

Today mood: 😊 😄 😎 🙂 😴 😵 😖

	Low	Medium	High
Energy level	☐	☐	☐
Sleep quality	☐	☐	☐
Stress level	☐	☐	☐
Activity level	☐	☐	☐

Today's goals:
- ☐ ....
- ☐ ....
- ☐ ....

Medications:
- ☐ ....
- ☐ ....
- ☐ ....

Supplements/Nutrition:
- ☐ ....
- ☐ ....
- ☐ ....

Water intake (1 cup = 8 oz)

Coffee I drank today

Juice I drank today

Meditation: from: .... to: .... total minutes: ....

Cardio: from: .... to: .... total calories burn: ....

Exercise: from: .... to: .... total minutes: ....
Type: ....

Daily events
- ☐ ....   ☐ ....
- ☐ ....   ☐ ....
- ☐ ....   ☐ ....

Daily important notes
....
....
....
....
....
....
....
....

DAILY FOOD LOG

Food	Amount	Cal	Protein	Carbs	Fats	Sugar
Breakfast time:..................						
Lunch time:..................						
Dinner time:..................						
Snacks time:..................						

FOOD TRIGGER TRACKER

Immediately after	After 1 hour	After 3 hours

Symptoms/Pains: ....
....
....
....
....
....
....

DAILY PROGRESS & TRACKER

Date: ....

Day: .... of my journey   Weight: ....   Mo - Tu - We - Th - Fr - Sa - Su

Daily affirmations: ....
....
....

	Low	Medium	High
Energy level	☐	☐	☐
Sleep quality	☐	☐	☐
Stress level	☐	☐	☐
Activity level	☐	☐	☐

Today mood: 😻 😊 😎 🙂 😴 😵 😠

Today's goals:
- ☐ ....
- ☐ ....
- ☐ ....

Medications:
- ☐ ....
- ☐ ....
- ☐ ....

Supplements/Nutrition:
- ☐ ....
- ☐ ....
- ☐ ....

Water intake (1 cup = 8 oz)

Coffee I drank today

Juice I drank today

Meditation: from: .... to: .... total minutes: ....

Cardio: from: .... to: .... total calories burn: ....

Exercise: from: .... to: .... total minutes: ....
Type: ....

Daily events
- ☐ ....
- ☐ ....
- ☐ ....
- ☐ ....
- ☐ ....
- ☐ ....

Daily important notes
....
....
....
....
....
....
....

DAILY FOOD LOG

Food	Amount	Cal	Protein	Carbs	Fats	Sugar
Breakfast time:.................						
Lunch time:.................						
Dinner time:.................						
Snacks time:.................						

FOOD TRIGGER TRACKER

Immediately after	After 1 hour	After 3 hours

Symptoms/Pains: ....
....
....
....
....
....
....
....

DAILY PROGRESS & TRACKER

Date: ....

Day:........... of my journey   Weight: ....

Mo - Tu - We - Th - Fr - Sa - Su

Daily affirmations: ....
....
....

Today mood: 😊 😄 😎 😐 😴 😵 😣

	Low	Medium	High
Energy level	☐	☐	☐
Sleep quality	☐	☐	☐
Stress level	☐	☐	☐
Activity level	☐	☐	☐

Today's goals:
- ☐ ....
- ☐ ....
- ☐ ....

Medications:
- ☐ ....
- ☐ ....
- ☐ ....

Supplements/Nutrition:
- ☐ ....
- ☐ ....
- ☐ ....

Water intake (1 cup = 8 oz)

Coffee I drank today

Juice I drank today

Meditation: from: .... to: .... total minutes: ....

Cardio: from: .... to: .... total calories burn: ....

Exercise: from: .... to: .... total minutes: ....
Type: ....

Daily events
- ☐ ....   ☐ ....
- ☐ ....   ☐ ....
- ☐ ....   ☐ ....

Daily important notes
....
....
....
....
....
....
....

DAILY FOOD LOG

Food	Amount	Cal	Protein	Carbs	Fats	Sugar
Breakfast time:..................						
Lunch time:..................						
Dinner time:..................						
Snacks time:						

FOOD TRIGGER TRACKER

Immediately after	After 1 hour	After 3 hours

Symptoms/Pains: ....
....
....
....
....
....
....

DAILY PROGRESS & TRACKER

Date: ....

Day: .... of my journey   Weight: ....

Mo - Tu - We - Th - Fr - Sa - Su

Daily affirmations: ....
....
....

	Low	Medium	High
Energy level	☐	☐	☐
Sleep quality	☐	☐	☐
Stress level	☐	☐	☐
Activity level	☐	☐	☐

Today mood: 😊 😄 😎 🙂 😴 😳 😕

Today's goals:
- ☐ ....
- ☐ ....
- ☐ ....

Water intake (1 cup = 8 oz)

Medications:
- ☐ ....
- ☐ ....
- ☐ ....

Coffee I drank today

Supplements/Nutrition:
- ☐ ....
- ☐ ....
- ☐ ....

Juice I drank today

Meditation: from: .... to: .... total minutes: ....

Cardio: from: .... to: .... total calories burn: ....

Exercise: from: .... to: .... total minutes: ....
Type: ....

Daily events
- ☐ ....
- ☐ ....
- ☐ ....
- ☐ ....
- ☐ ....
- ☐ ....

Daily important notes
....
....
....
....
....
....
....
....

DAILY FOOD LOG

Food	Amount	Cal	Protein	Carbs	Fats	Sugar
Breakfast time:.................						
Lunch time:.................						
Dinner time:.................						
Snacks time:.................						

FOOD TRIGGER TRACKER

Immediately after	After 1 hour	After 3 hours

Symptoms/Pains: ....
....
....
....
....
....
....

DAILY PROGRESS & TRACKER

Date: ....

Day: .... of my journey   Weight: ....   Mo - Tu - We - Th - Fr - Sa - Su

Daily affirmations: ....
....
....

Today mood: 😊 😄 😎 🙂 😴 🤒 😣

	Low	Medium	High
Energy level	☐	☐	☐
Sleep quality	☐	☐	☐
Stress level	☐	☐	☐
Activity level	☐	☐	☐

Today's goals:
☐ ....
☐ ....
☐ ....

Medications:
☐ ....
☐ ....
☐ ....

Supplements/Nutrition:
☐ ....
☐ ....
☐ ....

Water intake (1 cup = 8 oz)

Coffee I drank today

Juice I drank today

Meditation: from: .... to: .... total minutes: ....

Cardio: from: .... to: .... total calories burn: ....

Exercise: from: .... to: .... total minutes: ....
Type: ....

Daily events
☐ ....   ☐ ....
☐ ....   ☐ ....
☐ ....   ☐ ....

Daily important notes
....
....
....
....
....
....
....

DAILY FOOD LOG

Food	Amount	Cal	Protein	Carbs	Fats	Sugar
🍳 Breakfast time:						
🌐 Lunch time:						
🍽 Dinner time:						
🍿 Snacks time:						

FOOD TRIGGER TRACKER

Immediately after	After 1 hour	After 3 hours

Symptoms/Pains: ....
....
....
....
....
....
....

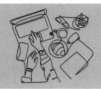

WEEKLY ACTIVITY PLANNER

WEEK OF: ....

WEEKLY CHALLENGES AND GOALS

- [ ] ....
- [ ] ....
- [ ] ....
- [ ] ....
- [ ] ....
- [ ] ....
- [ ] ....
- [ ] ....
- [ ] ....
- [ ] ....
- [ ] ....
- [ ] ....
- [ ] ....
- [ ] ....
- [ ] ....
- [ ] ....
- [ ] ....
- [ ] ....
- [ ] ....
- [ ] ....
- [ ] ....

WEEKLY TO-DO LISTS

- [ ] ....   - [ ] ....
- [ ] ....   - [ ] ....
- [ ] ....   - [ ] ....
- [ ] ....   - [ ] ....
- [ ] ....   - [ ] ....
- [ ] ....   - [ ] ....
- [ ] ....   - [ ] ....
- [ ] ....   - [ ] ....
- [ ] ....   - [ ] ....
- [ ] ....   - [ ] ....
- [ ] ....   - [ ] ....

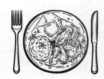

WEEKLY MEAL PLANNER

WEEK OF: ....

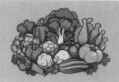

	BREAKFAST	SNACK	LUNCH	DINNER
MON				
TUE				
WED				
THU				
FRI				
SAT				
SUN				

DAILY PROGRESS & TRACKER

Date: ....

Day: .... of my journey   Weight: ....   Mo - Tu - We - Th - Fr - Sa - Su

Daily affirmations: ....
....
....

Today mood: 😊 😄 😎 🙂 😴 😵 😣

	Low	Medium	High
Energy level	☐	☐	☐
Sleep quality	☐	☐	☐
Stress level	☐	☐	☐
Activity level	☐	☐	☐

Today's goals:
☐ ....
☐ ....
☐ ....

Medications:
☐ ....
☐ ....
☐ ....

Supplements/Nutrition:
☐ ....
☐ ....
☐ ....

Water intake (1 cup = 8 oz)

Coffee I drank today

Juice I drank today

Meditation: from: .... to: .... total minutes: ....

Cardio: from: .... to: .... total calories burn: ....

Exercise: from: .... to: .... total minutes: ....
Type: ....

Daily events
☐ ....   ☐ ....
☐ ....   ☐ ....
☐ ....   ☐ ....

Daily important notes
....
....
....
....
....
....
....

DAILY FOOD LOG

Food	Amount	Cal	Protein	Carbs	Fats	Sugar
🍳 Breakfast time:..................						
🌐 Lunch time:..................						
🍳 Dinner time:..................						
🍿 Snacks time:..................						

FOOD TRIGGER TRACKER

Immediately after	After 1 hour	After 3 hours

Symptoms/Pains: ....
....
....
....
....
....
....
....

DAILY PROGRESS & TRACKER

Date: ....

Day: .... of my journey   Weight: ....

Mo - Tu - We - Th - Fr - Sa - Su

Daily affirmations: ....
....
....

Today mood: 😊 😄 😎 🙂 😴 😳 😖

	Low	Medium	High
Energy level	☐	☐	☐
Sleep quality	☐	☐	☐
Stress level	☐	☐	☐
Activity level	☐	☐	☐

Today's goals:
- ☐ ....
- ☐ ....
- ☐ ....

Medications:
- ☐ ....
- ☐ ....
- ☐ ....

Supplements/Nutrition:
- ☐ ....
- ☐ ....
- ☐ ....

Water intake (1 cup = 8 oz)

Coffee I drank today

Juice I drank today

Meditation: from: .... to: .... total minutes: ....

Cardio: from: .... to: .... total calories burn: ....

Exercise: from: .... to: .... total minutes: ....
Type: ....

Daily events
- ☐ ....
- ☐ ....
- ☐ ....
- ☐ ....
- ☐ ....
- ☐ ....

Daily important notes
....
....
....
....
....
....
....

DAILY FOOD LOG

Food	Amount	Cal	Protein	Carbs	Fats	Sugar
Breakfast time:....................						
Lunch time:....................						
Dinner time:....................						
Snacks time:						

FOOD TRIGGER TRACKER

Immediately after	After 1 hour	After 3 hours

Symptoms/Pains: ....
....
....
....
....
....
....

DAILY PROGRESS & TRACKER

Date: ....

Day: .... of my journey   Weight: ....   Mo - Tu - We - Th - Fr - Sa - Su

Daily affirmations: ....
....
....

Today mood: 😊 😄 😎 🙂 😴 😵 😣

	Low	Medium	High
Energy level	☐	☐	☐
Sleep quality	☐	☐	☐
Stress level	☐	☐	☐
Activity level	☐	☐	☐

Today's goals:
☐ ....
☐ ....
☐ ....

Medications:
☐ ....
☐ ....
☐ ....

Supplements/Nutrition:
☐ ....
☐ ....
☐ ....

Water intake (1 cup = 8 oz)

Coffee I drank today

Juice I drank today

Meditation: from: .... to: .... total minutes: ....

Cardio: from: .... to: .... total calories burn: ....

Exercise: from: .... to: .... total minutes: ....
Type: ....

Daily events
☐ ....   ☐ ....
☐ ....   ☐ ....
☐ ....   ☐ ....

Daily important notes
....
....
....
....
....
....
....

DAILY FOOD LOG

Food	Amount	Cal	Protein	Carbs	Fats	Sugar
Breakfast time:................						
Lunch time:.................						
Dinner time:.................						
Snacks time:..................						

FOOD TRIGGER TRACKER

Immediately after	After 1 hour	After 3 hours

Symptoms/Pains: ....
....
....
....
....
....
....
....

DAILY PROGRESS & TRACKER

Date: ....

Day:.......... of my journey   Weight: ....   Mo - Tu - We - Th - Fr - Sa - Su

Daily affirmations: ....
....
....

	Low	Medium	High
Energy level	☐	☐	☐
Sleep quality	☐	☐	☐
Stress level	☐	☐	☐
Activity level	☐	☐	☐

Today mood: 😊 😄 😎 🙂 😴 😵 😣

Today's goals:
☐ ....
☐ ....
☐ ....

Medications:
☐ ....
☐ ....
☐ ....

Supplements/Nutrition:
☐ ....
☐ ....
☐ ....

Water intake (1 cup = 8 oz)

Coffee I drank today

Juice I drank today

Meditation: from: .... to: .... total minutes: ....

Cardio: from: .... to: .... total calories burn:...........................

Exercise: from: ....to: ....total minutes: ....
Type: ....

Daily events
☐ ....   ☐ ....
☐ ....   ☐ ....
☐ ....   ☐ ....

Daily important notes
....
....
....
....
....
....
....

DAILY FOOD LOG

Food	Amount	Cal	Protein	Carbs	Fats	Sugar
Breakfast time:..................						
Lunch time:..................						
Dinner time:..................						
Snacks time:..................						

FOOD TRIGGER TRACKER

Immediately after	After 1 hour	After 3 hours

Symptoms/Pains: ....
....
....
....
....
....
....

DAILY PROGRESS & TRACKER

Date: ....

Day: .... of my journey   Weight: ....   Mo - Tu - We - Th - Fr - Sa - Su

Daily affirmations: ....
....
....

Today mood: 😊 😄 😎 🙂 😴 😳 😖

	Low	Medium	High
Energy level	☐	☐	☐
Sleep quality	☐	☐	☐
Stress level	☐	☐	☐
Activity level	☐	☐	☐

Today's goals:
- ☐ ....
- ☐ ....
- ☐ ....

Medications:
- ☐ ....
- ☐ ....
- ☐ ....

Supplements/Nutrition:
- ☐ ....
- ☐ ....
- ☐ ....

Water intake (1 cup = 8 oz)

Coffee I drank today

Juice I drank today

Meditation: from: .... to: .... total minutes: ....

Cardio: from: .... to: .... total calories burn: ....

Exercise: from: .... to: .... total minutes: ....
Type: ....

Daily events
- ☐ ....
- ☐ ....
- ☐ ....
- ☐ ....
- ☐ ....
- ☐ ....

Daily important notes
....
....
....
....
....
....
....

DAILY FOOD LOG

Food	Amount	Cal	Protein	Carbs	Fats	Sugar
Breakfast time:..................						
Lunch time:..................						
Dinner time:..................						
Snacks time:						

FOOD TRIGGER TRACKER

Immediately after	After 1 hour	After 3 hours

Symptoms/Pains: ....
....
....
....
....
....
....

DAILY PROGRESS & TRACKER

Date: ....

Day:.......... of my journey   Weight: ....

Mo - Tu - We - Th - Fr - Sa - Su

Daily affirmations: ....
....
....

	Low	Medium	High
Energy level	☐	☐	☐
Sleep quality	☐	☐	☐
Stress level	☐	☐	☐
Activity level	☐	☐	☐

Today mood: 😊 😀 😎 🙂 😴 😵 😖

Today's goals:
☐ ....
☐ ....
☐ ....

Medications:
☐ ....
☐ ....
☐ ....

Supplements/Nutrition:
☐ ....
☐ ....
☐ ....

Water intake (1 cup = 8 oz)

Coffee I drank today

Juice I drank today

Meditation: from: .... to: .... total minutes: ....

Cardio: from: .... to: .... total calories burn:..........................

Exercise: from: ....to: ....total minutes: ....
Type: ....

Daily events
☐ ....   ☐ ....
☐ ....   ☐ ....
☐ ....   ☐ ....

Daily important notes
....
....
....
....
....
....
....

DAILY FOOD LOG

Food	Amount	Cal	Protein	Carbs	Fats	Sugar
Breakfast time:.................						
Lunch time:.................						
Dinner time:.................						
Snacks time:.................						

FOOD TRIGGER TRACKER

Immediately after	After 1 hour	After 3 hours

Symptoms/Pains: ....
....
....
....
....
....
....

DAILY PROGRESS & TRACKER

Date: ....

Day: .... of my journey   Weight: ....   Mo - Tu - We - Th - Fr - Sa - Su

Daily affirmations: ....
....
....

Today mood: 😍 😊 😎 🙂 😴 🤢 😖

	Low	Medium	High
Energy level	☐	☐	☐
Sleep quality	☐	☐	☐
Stress level	☐	☐	☐
Activity level	☐	☐	☐

Today's goals:
☐ ....
☐ ....
☐ ....

Medications:
☐ ....
☐ ....
☐ ....

Supplements/Nutrition:
☐ ....
☐ ....
☐ ....

Water intake (1 cup = 8 oz)

Coffee I drank today

Juice I drank today

Meditation: from: .... to: .... total minutes: ....

Cardio: from: .... to: .... total calories burn: ....

Exercise: from: .... to: .... total minutes: ....
Type: ....

Daily events
☐ ....   ☐ ....
☐ ....   ☐ ....
☐ ....   ☐ ....

Daily important notes
....
....
....
....
....
....
....

DAILY FOOD LOG

Food	Amount	Cal	Protein	Carbs	Fats	Sugar
🍳 Breakfast time:.................						
🌐 Lunch time:.................						
🍽 Dinner time:.................						
🍿 Snacks time:.................						

FOOD TRIGGER TRACKER

Immediately after	After 1 hour	After 3 hours

Symptoms/Pains: ....
....
....
....
....
....
....

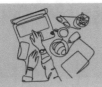

WEEKLY ACTIVITY PLANNER

WEEK OF: ....

WEEKLY CHALLENGES AND GOALS

- [ ] ....
- [ ] ....
- [ ] ....
- [ ] ....
- [ ] ....
- [ ] ....
- [ ] ....
- [ ] ....
- [ ] ....
- [ ] ....
- [ ] ....
- [ ] ....
- [ ] ....
- [ ] ....
- [ ] ....
- [ ] ....
- [ ] ....
- [ ] ....
- [ ] ....
- [ ] ....

WEEKLY TO-DO LISTS

- [ ] ....   - [ ] ....
- [ ] ....   - [ ] ....
- [ ] ....   - [ ] ....
- [ ] ....   - [ ] ....
- [ ] ....   - [ ] ....
- [ ] ....   - [ ] ....
- [ ] ....   - [ ] ....
- [ ] ....   - [ ] ....
- [ ] ....   - [ ] ....
- [ ] ....   - [ ] ....
- [ ] ....   - [ ] ....

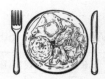 # WEEKLY MEAL PLANNER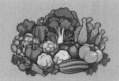

WEEK OF: ....

	BREAKFAST	SNACK	LUNCH	DINNER
MON				
TUE				
WED				
THU				
FRI				
SAT				
SUN				

DAILY PROGRESS & TRACKER

Date: ....

Day:............ of my journey   Weight: ....

Mo - Tu - We - Th - Fr - Sa - Su

Daily affirmations: ....
....
....

Today mood: 😊 😄 😎 🙂 😴 🤢 😌

	Low	Medium	High
Energy level	☐	☐	☐
Sleep quality	☐	☐	☐
Stress level	☐	☐	☐
Activity level	☐	☐	☐

Today's goals:
- ☐ ....
- ☐ ....
- ☐ ....

Medications:
- ☐ ....
- ☐ ....
- ☐ ....

Supplements/Nutrition:
- ☐ ....
- ☐ ....
- ☐ ....

Water intake (1 cup = 8 oz)

Coffee I drank today

Juice I drank today

Meditation: from: .... to: .... total minutes: ....

Cardio: from: .... to: .... total calories burn: ....

Exercise: from: .... to: .... total minutes: ....
Type: ....

Daily events
- ☐ ....
- ☐ ....
- ☐ ....
- ☐ ....
- ☐ ....
- ☐ ....

Daily important notes
....
....
....
....
....
....
....

DAILY FOOD LOG

Food	Amount	Cal	Protein	Carbs	Fats	Sugar
Breakfast time:................						
Lunch time:................						
Dinner time:................						
Snacks time:................						

FOOD TRIGGER TRACKER

Immediately after	After 1 hour	After 3 hours

Symptoms/Pains: ....
....
....
....
....
....
....

DAILY PROGRESS & TRACKER

Date: ....

Day:........... of my journey   Weight: ....

Mo - Tu - We - Th - Fr - Sa - Su

Daily affirmations: ....
....
....

Today mood: 😊 😄 😎 🙂 😴 😵 😖

	Low	Medium	High
Energy level	☐	☐	☐
Sleep quality	☐	☐	☐
Stress level	☐	☐	☐
Activity level	☐	☐	☐

Today's goals:
- ☐ ....
- ☐ ....
- ☐ ....

Medications:
- ☐ ....
- ☐ ....
- ☐ ....

Supplements/Nutrition:
- ☐ ....
- ☐ ....
- ☐ ....

Water intake (1 cup = 8 oz)

Coffee I drank today

Juice I drank today

Meditation: from: .... to: .... total minutes: ....

Cardio: from: .... to: .... total calories burn:.........................

Exercise: from: .... to: .... total minutes: ....
Type: ....

Daily events
- ☐ ....
- ☐ ....
- ☐ ....
- ☐ ....
- ☐ ....
- ☐ ....

Daily important notes
....
....
....
....
....
....
....

DAILY FOOD LOG

Food	Amount	Cal	Protein	Carbs	Fats	Sugar
🍳 Breakfast time:..................						
🌍 Lunch time:..................						
🍳 Dinner time:..................						
🍪 Snacks time:..................						

FOOD TRIGGER TRACKER

Immediately after	After 1 hour	After 3 hours

Symptoms/Pains: ....
....
....
....
....
....
....
....

DAILY PROGRESS & TRACKER

Date: ....

Day: .... of my journey   Weight: ....   Mo - Tu - We - Th - Fr - Sa - Su

Daily affirmations: ....
....
....

Today mood: 😊 😄 😎 🙂 😴 😵 😖

	Low	Medium	High
Energy level	☐	☐	☐
Sleep quality	☐	☐	☐
Stress level	☐	☐	☐
Activity level	☐	☐	☐

Today's goals:
- ☐ ....
- ☐ ....
- ☐ ....

Medications:
- ☐ ....
- ☐ ....
- ☐ ....

Supplements/Nutrition:
- ☐ ....
- ☐ ....
- ☐ ....

Water intake (1 cup = 8 oz)

Coffee I drank today

Juice I drank today

Meditation: from: .... to: .... total minutes: ....

Cardio: from: .... to: .... total calories burn: ....

Exercise: from: .... to: .... total minutes: ....
Type: ....

Daily events
- ☐ .... ☐ ....
- ☐ .... ☐ ....
- ☐ .... ☐ ....

Daily important notes
....
....
....
....
....
....
....

DAILY FOOD LOG

Food	Amount	Cal	Protein	Carbs	Fats	Sugar
Breakfast time:.................						
Lunch time:.................						
Dinner time:.................						
Snacks time:.................						

FOOD TRIGGER TRACKER

Immediately after	After 1 hour	After 3 hours

Symptoms/Pains: ....
....
....
....
....
....
....

DAILY PROGRESS & TRACKER

Date: ....

Day: .... of my journey   Weight: ....

Mo - Tu - We - Th - Fr - Sa - Su

Daily affirmations: ....
....
....

	Low	Medium	High
Energy level	☐	☐	☐
Sleep quality	☐	☐	☐
Stress level	☐	☐	☐
Activity level	☐	☐	☐

Today mood: 😊 😄 😎 🙂 😴 🤪 😵

Today's goals:

☐ ....
☐ ....
☐ ....

Medications:

☐ ....
☐ ....
☐ ....

Supplements/Nutrition:

☐ ....
☐ ....
☐ ....

Water intake (1 cup = 8 oz)

Coffee I drank today

Juice I drank today

Meditation: from: .... to: .... total minutes: ....

Cardio: from: .... to: .... total calories burn: ....

Exercise: from: .... to: .... total minutes: ....
Type: ....

Daily events

☐ ....   ☐ ....
☐ ....   ☐ ....
☐ ....   ☐ ....

Daily important notes

....
....
....
....
....
....
....

DAILY FOOD LOG

Food	Amount	Cal	Protein	Carbs	Fats	Sugar
Breakfast time:...............						
Lunch time:...............						
Dinner time:...............						
Snacks time:...............						

FOOD TRIGGER TRACKER

Immediately after	After 1 hour	After 3 hours

Symptoms/Pains: ....
....
....
....
....
....
....

DAILY PROGRESS & TRACKER

Date: ....

Day: .... of my journey   Weight: ....   Mo - Tu - We - Th - Fr - Sa - Su

Daily affirmations: ....
....
....

Today mood: 😄 😊 😎 🙂 😴 😵 😖

	Low	Medium	High
Energy level	☐	☐	☐
Sleep quality	☐	☐	☐
Stress level	☐	☐	☐
Activity level	☐	☐	☐

Today's goals:
☐ ....
☐ ....
☐ ....

Medications:
☐ ....
☐ ....
☐ ....

Supplements/Nutrition:
☐ ....
☐ ....
☐ ....

Water intake (1 cup = 8 oz)

Coffee I drank today

Juice I drank today

Meditation: from: .... to: .... total minutes: ....

Cardio: from: .... to: .... total calories burn: ....

Exercise: from: .... to: .... total minutes: ....
Type: ....

Daily events
☐ ....   ☐ ....
☐ ....   ☐ ....
☐ ....   ☐ ....

Daily important notes
....
....
....
....
....
....
....
....

DAILY FOOD LOG

Food	Amount	Cal	Protein	Carbs	Fats	Sugar
Breakfast time:................						
Lunch time:................						
Dinner time:................						
Snacks time:						

FOOD TRIGGER TRACKER

Immediately after	After 1 hour	After 3 hours

Symptoms/Pains: ....
....
....
....
....
....
....

DAILY PROGRESS & TRACKER

Date: ....

Day:........... of my journey   Weight: ....

Mo - Tu - We - Th - Fr - Sa - Su

Daily affirmations: ....
....
....

Today mood: 😊 😀 😎 🙂 😴 😵 😖

	Low	Medium	High
Energy level	☐	☐	☐
Sleep quality	☐	☐	☐
Stress level	☐	☐	☐
Activity level	☐	☐	☐

Today's goals:
- ☐ ....
- ☐ ....
- ☐ ....

Medications:
- ☐ ....
- ☐ ....
- ☐ ....

Supplements/Nutrition:
- ☐ ....
- ☐ ....
- ☐ ....

Water intake (1 cup = 8 oz)

Coffee I drank today

Juice I drank today

Meditation: from: .... to: .... total minutes: ....

Cardio: from: .... to: .... total calories burn: ....

Exercise: from: .... to: .... total minutes: ....
Type: ....

Daily events
- ☐ ....
- ☐ ....
- ☐ ....
- ☐ ....
- ☐ ....
- ☐ ....

Daily important notes
....
....
....
....
....
....
....

DAILY FOOD LOG

Food	Amount	Cal	Protein	Carbs	Fats	Sugar
Breakfast time:................						
Lunch time:................						
Dinner time:................						
Snacks time:................						

FOOD TRIGGER TRACKER

Immediately after	After 1 hour	After 3 hours

Symptoms/Pains: ....
....
....
....
....
....

DAILY PROGRESS & TRACKER

Date: ....

Day: .... of my journey   Weight: ....   Mo - Tu - We - Th - Fr - Sa - Su

Daily affirmations: ....
....
....

Today mood: 😆 😊 😎 🙂 😴 😵 😣

	Low	Medium	High
Energy level	☐	☐	☐
Sleep quality	☐	☐	☐
Stress level	☐	☐	☐
Activity level	☐	☐	☐

Today's goals:
- ☐ ....
- ☐ ....
- ☐ ....

Medications:
- ☐ ....
- ☐ ....
- ☐ ....

Supplements/Nutrition:
- ☐ ....
- ☐ ....
- ☐ ....

Water intake (1 cup = 8 oz)

Coffee I drank today

Juice I drank today

Meditation: from: .... to: .... total minutes: ....

Cardio: from: .... to: .... total calories burn: ....

Exercise: from: .... to: .... total minutes: ....
Type: ....

Daily events
- ☐ ....   ☐ ....
- ☐ ....   ☐ ....
- ☐ ....   ☐ ....

Daily important notes
....
....
....
....
....
....
....
....

DAILY FOOD LOG

Food	Amount	Cal	Protein	Carbs	Fats	Sugar
Breakfast time:................						
Lunch time:................						
Dinner time:................						
Snacks time:................						

FOOD TRIGGER TRACKER

Immediately after	After 1 hour	After 3 hours

Symptoms/Pains: ....
....
....
....
....
....

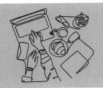

WEEKLY ACTIVITY PLANNER

WEEK OF: ....

WEEKLY CHALLENGES AND GOALS

- [ ] ....
- [ ] ....
- [ ] ....
- [ ] ....
- [ ] ....
- [ ] ....
- [ ] ....
- [ ] ....
- [ ] ....
- [ ] ....
- [ ] ....
- [ ] ....
- [ ] ....
- [ ] ....
- [ ] ....
- [ ] ....
- [ ] ....
- [ ] ....

WEEKLY TO-DO LISTS

- [ ] ....   - [ ] ....
- [ ] ....   - [ ] ....
- [ ] ....   - [ ] ....
- [ ] ....   - [ ] ....
- [ ] ....   - [ ] ....
- [ ] ....   - [ ] ....
- [ ] ....   - [ ] ....
- [ ] ....   - [ ] ....
- [ ] ....   - [ ] ....
- [ ] ....   - [ ] ....
- [ ] ....   - [ ] ....
- [ ] ....   - [ ] ....

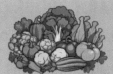

WEEKLY MEAL PLANNER

WEEK OF: ....

	BREAKFAST	SNACK	LUNCH	DINNER
MON				
TUE				
WED				
THU				
FRI				
SAT				
SUN				

DAILY PROGRESS & TRACKER

Date: ....

Day: .... of my journey   Weight: ....

Mo - Tu - We - Th - Fr - Sa - Su

Daily affirmations: ....
....
....

Today mood: 😊 😁 😎 😐 😴 😵 😖

	Low	Medium	High
Energy level	☐	☐	☐
Sleep quality	☐	☐	☐
Stress level	☐	☐	☐
Activity level	☐	☐	☐

Today's goals:
☐ ....
☐ ....
☐ ....

Water intake (1 cup = 8 oz)

Medications:
☐ ....
☐ ....
☐ ....

Coffee I drank today

Supplements/Nutrition:
☐ ....
☐ ....
☐ ....

Juice I drank today

Meditation: from: .... to: .... total minutes: ....

Cardio: from: .... to: .... total calories burn: ....

Exercise: from: .... to: .... total minutes: ....
Type: ....

Daily events
☐ ....   ☐ ....
☐ ....   ☐ ....
☐ ....   ☐ ....

Daily important notes
....
....
....
....
....
....
....

DAILY FOOD LOG

Food	Amount	Cal	Protein	Carbs	Fats	Sugar
Breakfast time:..................						
Lunch time:..................						
Dinner time:..................						
Snacks time:..................						

FOOD TRIGGER TRACKER

Immediately after	After 1 hour	After 3 hours

Symptoms/Pains: ....

....

....

....

....

....

....

DAILY PROGRESS & TRACKER

Date: ....

Day:.......... of my journey   Weight: ....

Mo - Tu - We - Th - Fr - Sa - Su

Daily affirmations: ....
....
....

	Low	Medium	High
Energy level	☐	☐	☐
Sleep quality	☐	☐	☐
Stress level	☐	☐	☐
Activity level	☐	☐	☐

Today mood: 😊 😄 😎 🙂 😴 😵 😣

Today's goals:
☐ ....
☐ ....
☐ ....

Medications:
☐ ....
☐ ....
☐ ....

Supplements/Nutrition:
☐ ....
☐ ....
☐ ....

Water intake (1 cup = 8 oz)

Coffee I drank today

Juice I drank today

Meditation: from: .... to: .... total minutes: ....

Cardio: from: .... to: .... total calories burn: ....

Exercise: from: .... to: .... total minutes: ....
Type: ....

Daily events
☐ ....   ☐ ....
☐ ....   ☐ ....
☐ ....   ☐ ....

Daily important notes
....
....
....
....
....
....
....

DAILY FOOD LOG

Food	Amount	Cal	Protein	Carbs	Fats	Sugar
Breakfast time:...................						
Lunch time:...................						
Dinner time:...................						
Snacks time:						

FOOD TRIGGER TRACKER

Immediately after	After 1 hour	After 3 hours

Symptoms/Pains: ....

....

....

....

....

....

....

DAILY PROGRESS & TRACKER

Date: ....

Day: .... of my journey   Weight: ....

Mo - Tu - We - Th - Fr - Sa - Su

Daily affirmations: ....
....
....

Today mood: 😊 😄 😎 🙂 😴 😵 😕

	Low	Medium	High
Energy level	☐	☐	☐
Sleep quality	☐	☐	☐
Stress level	☐	☐	☐
Activity level	☐	☐	☐

Today's goals:
- ☐ ....
- ☐ ....
- ☐ ....

Medications:
- ☐ ....
- ☐ ....
- ☐ ....

Supplements/Nutrition:
- ☐ ....
- ☐ ....
- ☐ ....

Water intake (1 cup = 8 oz)

Coffee I drank today

Juice I drank today

Meditation: from: .... to: .... total minutes: ....

Cardio: from: .... to: .... total calories burn: ....

Exercise: from: .... to: .... total minutes: ....
Type: ....

Daily events
- ☐ ....
- ☐ ....
- ☐ ....
- ☐ ....
- ☐ ....
- ☐ ....

Daily important notes
....
....
....
....
....
....
....
....

DAILY FOOD LOG

Food	Amount	Cal	Protein	Carbs	Fats	Sugar
🍳 Breakfast time:..................						
🌍 Lunch time:..................						
🍽 Dinner time:..................						
🍿 Snacks time:..................						

FOOD TRIGGER TRACKER

Immediately after	After 1 hour	After 3 hours

Symptoms/Pains: ....
....
....
....
....
....
....
....

DAILY PROGRESS & TRACKER

Date: ....

Day: .... of my journey   Weight: ....

Mo - Tu - We - Th - Fr - Sa - Su

Daily affirmations: ....
....
....

Today mood: 😊 😄 😎 🙂 😴 😵 😖

	Low	Medium	High
Energy level	☐	☐	☐
Sleep quality	☐	☐	☐
Stress level	☐	☐	☐
Activity level	☐	☐	☐

Today's goals:
☐ ....
☐ ....
☐ ....

Medications:
☐ ....
☐ ....
☐ ....

Supplements/Nutrition:
☐ ....
☐ ....
☐ ....

Water intake (1 cup = 8 oz)

Coffee I drank today

Juice I drank today

Meditation: from: .... to: .... total minutes: ....

Cardio: from: .... to: .... total calories burn: ....

Exercise: from: .... to: .... total minutes: ....
Type: ....

Daily events
☐ ....   ☐ ....
☐ ....   ☐ ....
☐ ....   ☐ ....

Daily important notes
....
....
....
....
....
....
....

DAILY FOOD LOG

Food	Amount	Cal	Protein	Carbs	Fats	Sugar
🍳 Breakfast time:..................						
🌍 Lunch time:..................						
🍳 Dinner time:..................						
🍿 Snacks time:..................						

FOOD TRIGGER TRACKER

Immediately after	After 1 hour	After 3 hours

Symptoms/Pains: ....
....
....
....
....
....
....

DAILY PROGRESS & TRACKER

Date: ....

Day: .... of my journey   Weight: ....   Mo - Tu - We - Th - Fr - Sa - Su

Daily affirmations: ....
....
....

Today mood: 😊 😄 😎 🙂 😴 🤪 😣

	Low	Medium	High
Energy level	☐	☐	☐
Sleep quality	☐	☐	☐
Stress level	☐	☐	☐
Activity level	☐	☐	☐

Today's goals:
- ☐ ....
- ☐ ....
- ☐ ....

Medications:
- ☐ ....
- ☐ ....
- ☐ ....

Supplements/Nutrition:
- ☐ ....
- ☐ ....
- ☐ ....

Water intake (1 cup = 8 oz)

Coffee I drank today

Juice I drank today

Meditation: from: .... to: .... total minutes: ....

Cardio: from: .... to: .... total calories burn: ....

Exercise: from: .... to: .... total minutes: ....
Type: ....

Daily events
- ☐ ....
- ☐ ....
- ☐ ....
- ☐ ....
- ☐ ....
- ☐ ....

Daily important notes
....
....
....
....
....
....
....

DAILY FOOD LOG

Food	Amount	Cal	Protein	Carbs	Fats	Sugar
Breakfast time:..................						
Lunch time:..................						
Dinner time:..................						
Snacks time:..................						

FOOD TRIGGER TRACKER

Immediately after	After 1 hour	After 3 hours

Symptoms/Pains: ....
....
....
....
....
....
....

DAILY PROGRESS & TRACKER

Date: ....

Day:.......... of my journey   Weight: ....   Mo - Tu - We - Th - Fr - Sa - Su

Daily affirmations: ....
....
....

	Low	Medium	High
Energy level	☐	☐	☐
Sleep quality	☐	☐	☐
Stress level	☐	☐	☐
Activity level	☐	☐	☐

Today mood: 😊 😄 😎 🙂 😴 😵 😣

Today's goals:
- ☐ ....
- ☐ ....
- ☐ ....

Water intake (1 cup = 8 oz)

Medications:
- ☐ ....
- ☐ ....
- ☐ ....

Coffee I drank today

Supplements/Nutrition:
- ☐ ....
- ☐ ....
- ☐ ....

Juice I drank today

Meditation: from: .... to: .... total minutes: ....

Cardio: from: .... to: .... total calories burn:........................

Exercise: from: .... to: .... total minutes: ....
Type: ....

Daily events
- ☐ .... ☐ ....
- ☐ .... ☐ ....
- ☐ .... ☐ ....

Daily important notes
....
....
....
....
....
....
....

DAILY FOOD LOG

Food	Amount	Cal	Protein	Carbs	Fats	Sugar
Breakfast time:..................						
Lunch time:..................						
Dinner time:..................						
Snacks time:..................						

FOOD TRIGGER TRACKER

Immediately after	After 1 hour	After 3 hours

Symptoms/Pains: ....
....
....
....
....
....
....

DAILY PROGRESS & TRACKER

Date: ....

Day: .... of my journey   Weight: ....   Mo - Tu - We - Th - Fr - Sa - Su

Daily affirmations: ....
....
....

	Low	Medium	High
Energy level	☐	☐	☐
Sleep quality	☐	☐	☐
Stress level	☐	☐	☐
Activity level	☐	☐	☐

Today mood: 😊 ☺ 😎 🙂 😴 😵 😖

Today's goals:
- ☐ ....
- ☐ ....
- ☐ ....

Medications:
- ☐ ....
- ☐ ....
- ☐ ....

Supplements/Nutrition:
- ☐ ....
- ☐ ....
- ☐ ....

Water intake (1 cup = 8 oz)

Coffee I drank today

Juice I drank today

Meditation: from: .... to: .... total minutes: ....

Cardio: from: .... to: .... total calories burn: ....

Exercise: from: .... to: .... total minutes: ....
Type: ....

Daily events
- ☐ .... ☐ ....
- ☐ .... ☐ ....
- ☐ .... ☐ ....

Daily important notes
....
....
....
....
....
....
....
....

DAILY FOOD LOG

Food	Amount	Cal	Protein	Carbs	Fats	Sugar
Breakfast time:................						
Lunch time:................						
Dinner time:................						
Snacks time:................						

FOOD TRIGGER TRACKER

Immediately after	After 1 hour	After 3 hours

Symptoms/Pains: ....
....
....
....
....
....
....

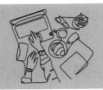

WEEKLY ACTIVITY PLANNER

WEEK OF: ....

WEEKLY CHALLENGES AND GOALS

- [ ] ....
- [ ] ....
- [ ] ....
- [ ] ....
- [ ] ....
- [ ] ....
- [ ] ....
- [ ] ....
- [ ] ....
- [ ] ....
- [ ] ....
- [ ] ....
- [ ] ....
- [ ] ....
- [ ] ....
- [ ] ....
- [ ] ....
- [ ] ....

WEEKLY TO-DO LISTS

- [ ] ....   - [ ] ....
- [ ] ....   - [ ] ....
- [ ] ....   - [ ] ....
- [ ] ....   - [ ] ....
- [ ] ....   - [ ] ....
- [ ] ....   - [ ] ....
- [ ] ....   - [ ] ....
- [ ] ....   - [ ] ....
- [ ] ....   - [ ] ....
- [ ] ....   - [ ] ....
- [ ] ....   - [ ] ....
- [ ] ....   - [ ] ....

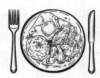 # WEEKLY MEAL PLANNER

WEEK OF: ....

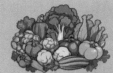

	BREAKFAST	SNACK	LUNCH	DINNER
MON				
TUE				
WED				
THU				
FRI				
SAT				
SUN				

DAILY PROGRESS & TRACKER

Date: ....

Day: .... of my journey   Weight: ....   Mo - Tu - We - Th - Fr - Sa - Su

| Daily affirmations: .... |
| .... |
| .... |

	Low	Medium	High
Energy level	☐	☐	☐
Sleep quality	☐	☐	☐
Stress level	☐	☐	☐
Activity level	☐	☐	☐

Today mood: 😊 😄 😎 😐 😴 😵 😖

Today's goals:
- ☐ ....
- ☐ ....
- ☐ ....

Medications:
- ☐ ....
- ☐ ....
- ☐ ....

Supplements/Nutrition:
- ☐ ....
- ☐ ....
- ☐ ....

Water intake (1 cup = 8 oz)

Coffee I drank today

Juice I drank today

Meditation: from: .... to: .... total minutes: ....

Cardio: from: .... to: .... total calories burn: ....

Exercise: from: .... to: .... total minutes: ....
Type: ....

Daily events
- ☐ ....   ☐ ....
- ☐ ....   ☐ ....
- ☐ ....   ☐ ....

Daily important notes
....
....
....
....
....
....

DAILY FOOD LOG

Food	Amount	Cal	Protein	Carbs	Fats	Sugar
Breakfast time:....................						
Lunch time:....................						
Dinner time:....................						
Snacks time:....................						

FOOD TRIGGER TRACKER

Immediately after	After 1 hour	After 3 hours

Symptoms/Pains: ....

....

....

....

....

....

....

....

DAILY PROGRESS & TRACKER

Date: ....

Day: .... of my journey   Weight: ....

Mo - Tu - We - Th - Fr - Sa - Su

Daily affirmations: ....
....
....

	Low	Medium	High
Energy level	☐	☐	☐
Sleep quality	☐	☐	☐
Stress level	☐	☐	☐
Activity level	☐	☐	☐

Today mood: 😊 😁 😎 🙂 😴 🤪 😕

Today's goals:
- ☐ ....
- ☐ ....
- ☐ ....

Medications:
- ☐ ....
- ☐ ....
- ☐ ....

Supplements/Nutrition:
- ☐ ....
- ☐ ....
- ☐ ....

Water intake (1 cup = 8 oz)

Coffee I drank today

Juice I drank today

Meditation: from: .... to: .... total minutes: ....

Cardio: from: .... to: .... total calories burn: ....

Exercise: from: .... to: .... total minutes: ....
Type: ....

Daily events
- ☐ ....
- ☐ ....
- ☐ ....
- ☐ ....
- ☐ ....
- ☐ ....

Daily important notes
....
....
....
....
....
....
....

DAILY FOOD LOG

Food	Amount	Cal	Protein	Carbs	Fats	Sugar
Breakfast time:..................						
Lunch time:..................						
Dinner time:..................						
Snacks time:..................						

FOOD TRIGGER TRACKER

Immediately after	After 1 hour	After 3 hours

Symptoms/Pains: ....
....
....
....
....
....
....

DAILY PROGRESS & TRACKER

Date: ....

Day:.......... of my journey   Weight: ....   Mo - Tu - We - Th - Fr - Sa - Su

Daily affirmations: ....
....
....

Today mood: 😊 😄 😎 😐 😴 😵 😌

	Low	Medium	High
Energy level	☐	☐	☐
Sleep quality	☐	☐	☐
Stress level	☐	☐	☐
Activity level	☐	☐	☐

Today's goals:
☐ ....
☐ ....
☐ ....

Medications:
☐ ....
☐ ....
☐ ....

Supplements/Nutrition:
☐ ....
☐ ....
☐ ....

Water intake (1 cup = 8 oz)

Coffee I drank today

Juice I drank today

Meditation: from: .... to: .... total minutes: ....

Cardio: from: .... to: .... total calories burn: ....

Exercise: from: .... to: .... total minutes: ....
Type: ....

Daily events
☐ ....   ☐ ....
☐ ....   ☐ ....
☐ ....   ☐ ....

Daily important notes
....
....
....
....
....
....
....

DAILY FOOD LOG

Food	Amount	Cal	Protein	Carbs	Fats	Sugar
🍳 Breakfast time:................						
🌍 Lunch time:................						
🍛 Dinner time:................						
🍪 Snacks time:................						

FOOD TRIGGER TRACKER

Immediately after	After 1 hour	After 3 hours

Symptoms/Pains: ....
....
....
....
....
....
....

DAILY PROGRESS & TRACKER

Date: ....

Day: .... of my journey   Weight: ....   Mo - Tu - We - Th - Fr - Sa - Su

Daily affirmations: ....
....
....

	Low	Medium	High
Energy level	☐	☐	☐
Sleep quality	☐	☐	☐
Stress level	☐	☐	☐
Activity level	☐	☐	☐

Today mood: 😄 😊 😎 🙂 😴 😵 😖

Today's goals:
☐ ....
☐ ....
☐ ....

Medications:
☐ ....
☐ ....
☐ ....

Supplements/Nutrition:
☐ ....
☐ ....
☐ ....

Water intake (1 cup = 8 oz)

Coffee I drank today

Juice I drank today

Meditation: from: .... to: .... total minutes: ....

Cardio: from: .... to: .... total calories burn: ....

Exercise: from: .... to: .... total minutes: ....
Type: ....

Daily events
☐ ....   ☐ ....
☐ ....   ☐ ....
☐ ....   ☐ ....

Daily important notes
....
....
....
....
....
....
....

DAILY FOOD LOG

Food	Amount	Cal	Protein	Carbs	Fats	Sugar
Breakfast time:..................						
Lunch time:..................						
Dinner time:..................						
Snacks time:..................						

FOOD TRIGGER TRACKER

Immediately after	After 1 hour	After 3 hours

Symptoms/Pains: ....
....
....
....
....
....
....

DAILY PROGRESS & TRACKER

Date: ....

Day:.......... of my journey   Weight: ....   Mo - Tu - We - Th - Fr - Sa - Su

Daily affirmations: ....
....
....

Today mood: 😊 😄 😎 😐 😴 😵 😔

	Low	Medium	High
Energy level	☐	☐	☐
Sleep quality	☐	☐	☐
Stress level	☐	☐	☐
Activity level	☐	☐	☐

Today's goals:
☐ ....
☐ ....
☐ ....

Medications:
☐ ....
☐ ....
☐ ....

Supplements/Nutrition:
☐ ....
☐ ....
☐ ....

Water intake (1 cup = 8 oz)

Coffee I drank today

Juice I drank today

Meditation: from: .... to: .... total minutes: ....

Cardio: from: .... to: .... total calories burn:........................

Exercise: from: .... to: .... total minutes: ....
Type: ....

Daily events
☐ ....   ☐ ....
☐ ....   ☐ ....
☐ ....   ☐ ....

Daily important notes
....
....
....
....
....
....
....

DAILY FOOD LOG

Food	Amount	Cal	Protein	Carbs	Fats	Sugar
Breakfast time:.................						
Lunch time:.................						
Dinner time:.................						
Snacks time:.................						

FOOD TRIGGER TRACKER

Immediately after	After 1 hour	After 3 hours

Symptoms/Pains: ....
....
....
....
....
....
....

DAILY PROGRESS & TRACKER

Date: ....

Day: .... of my journey   Weight: ....

Mo - Tu - We - Th - Fr - Sa - Su

Daily affirmations: ....
....
....

Today mood: 😊 😁 😎 😐 😴 😵 😟

	Low	Medium	High
Energy level	☐	☐	☐
Sleep quality	☐	☐	☐
Stress level	☐	☐	☐
Activity level	☐	☐	☐

Today's goals:
☐ ....
☐ ....
☐ ....

Medications:
☐ ....
☐ ....
☐ ....

Supplements/Nutrition:
☐ ....
☐ ....
☐ ....

Water intake (1 cup = 8 oz)

Coffee I drank today

Juice I drank today

Meditation: from: .... to: .... total minutes: ....

Cardio: from: .... to: .... total calories burn: ....

Exercise: from: .... to: .... total minutes: ....
Type: ....

Daily events
☐ ....   ☐ ....
☐ ....   ☐ ....
☐ ....   ☐ ....

Daily important notes
....
....
....
....
....
....
....

DAILY FOOD LOG

Food	Amount	Cal	Protein	Carbs	Fats	Sugar
Breakfast time:.................						
Lunch time:.................						
Dinner time:.................						
Snacks time:.................						

FOOD TRIGGER TRACKER

Immediately after	After 1 hour	After 3 hours

Symptoms/Pains: ....
....
....
....
....
....
....

DAILY PROGRESS & TRACKER

Date: ....

Day:............ of my journey   Weight: ....   Mo - Tu - We - Th - Fr - Sa - Su

Daily affirmations: ....
....
....

Today mood: 😊 😁 😎 😐 😴 😵 😖

	Low	Medium	High
Energy level	☐	☐	☐
Sleep quality	☐	☐	☐
Stress level	☐	☐	☐
Activity level	☐	☐	☐

Today's goals:
☐ ....
☐ ....
☐ ....

Medications:
☐ ....
☐ ....
☐ ....

Supplements/Nutrition:
☐ ....
☐ ....
☐ ....

Water intake (1 cup = 8 oz)

Coffee I drank today

Juice I drank today

Meditation: from: .... to: .... total minutes: ....

Cardio: from: .... to: .... total calories burn: ....

Exercise: from: .... to: .... total minutes: ....
Type: ....

Daily events
☐ ....   ☐ ....
☐ ....   ☐ ....
☐ ....   ☐ ....

Daily important notes
....
....
....
....
....
....
....

DAILY FOOD LOG

Food	Amount	Cal	Protein	Carbs	Fats	Sugar
Breakfast time:.................						
Lunch time:.................						
Dinner time:.................						
Snacks time:.................						

FOOD TRIGGER TRACKER

Immediately after	After 1 hour	After 3 hours

Symptoms/Pains: ....
....
....
....
....
....
....
....

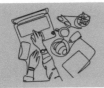

WEEKLY ACTIVITY PLANNER

WEEK OF: ....

WEEKLY CHALLENGES AND GOALS

- [ ] ....
- [ ] ....
- [ ] ....
- [ ] ....
- [ ] ....
- [ ] ....
- [ ] ....
- [ ] ....
- [ ] ....
- [ ] ....
- [ ] ....
- [ ] ....
- [ ] ....
- [ ] ....
- [ ] ....
- [ ] ....
- [ ] ....
- [ ] ....
- [ ] ....
- [ ] ....

WEEKLY TO-DO LISTS

- [ ] ....
- [ ] ....
- [ ] ....
- [ ] ....
- [ ] ....
- [ ] ....
- [ ] ....
- [ ] ....
- [ ] ....
- [ ] ....
- [ ] ....
- [ ] ....

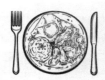

WEEKLY MEAL PLANNER

WEEK OF: ....

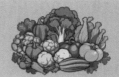

	BREAKFAST	SNACK	LUNCH	DINNER
MON				
TUE				
WED				
THU				
FRI				
SAT				
SUN				

DAILY PROGRESS & TRACKER

Date: ....

Day:.......... of my journey   Weight: ....   Mo - Tu - We - Th - Fr - Sa - Su

Daily affirmations: ....
....
....

Today mood: 😊 😁 😎 😐 😴 😵 😖

	Low	Medium	High
Energy level	☐	☐	☐
Sleep quality	☐	☐	☐
Stress level	☐	☐	☐
Activity level	☐	☐	☐

Today's goals:
☐ ....
☐ ....
☐ ....

Medications:
☐ ....
☐ ....
☐ ....

Supplements/Nutrition:
☐ ....
☐ ....
☐ ....

Water intake (1 cup = 8 oz)

Coffee I drank today

Juice I drank today

Meditation: from: .... to: .... total minutes: ....

Cardio: from: .... to: .... total calories burn:.........................

Exercise: from: .... to: .... total minutes: ....
Type: ....

Daily events
☐ ....   ☐ ....
☐ ....   ☐ ....
☐ ....   ☐ ....

Daily important notes
....
....
....
....
....
....
....

DAILY FOOD LOG

Food	Amount	Cal	Protein	Carbs	Fats	Sugar
Breakfast time:..................						
Lunch time:..................						
Dinner time:..................						
Snacks time:..................						

FOOD TRIGGER TRACKER

Immediately after	After 1 hour	After 3 hours

Symptoms/Pains: ....

....

....

....

....

....

....

DAILY PROGRESS & TRACKER

Date: ....

Day: .... of my journey   Weight: ....   Mo - Tu - We - Th - Fr - Sa - Su

Daily affirmations: ....
....
....

Today mood: 😊 😃 😎 🙂 😴 😵 😣

	Low	Medium	High
Energy level	☐	☐	☐
Sleep quality	☐	☐	☐
Stress level	☐	☐	☐
Activity level	☐	☐	☐

Today's goals:
- ☐ ....
- ☐ ....
- ☐ ....

Medications:
- ☐ ....
- ☐ ....
- ☐ ....

Supplements/Nutrition:
- ☐ ....
- ☐ ....
- ☐ ....

Water intake (1 cup = 8 oz)

Coffee I drank today

Juice I drank today

Meditation: from: .... to: .... total minutes: ....

Cardio: from: .... to: .... total calories burn: ....

Exercise: from: .... to: .... total minutes: ....
Type: ....

Daily events
- ☐ ....
- ☐ ....
- ☐ ....
- ☐ ....
- ☐ ....
- ☐ ....

Daily important notes
....
....
....
....
....
....
....

DAILY FOOD LOG

Food	Amount	Cal	Protein	Carbs	Fats	Sugar
Breakfast time:..................						
Lunch time:..................						
Dinner time:..................						
Snacks time:..................						

FOOD TRIGGER TRACKER

Immediately after	After 1 hour	After 3 hours

Symptoms/Pains: ....

....

....

....

....

....

....

DAILY PROGRESS & TRACKER

Date: ....

Day: .... of my journey   Weight: ....   Mo - Tu - We - Th - Fr - Sa - Su

Daily affirmations: ....
....
....

Today mood: 😊 😄 😎 😐 😴 😵 😖

	Low	Medium	High
Energy level	☐	☐	☐
Sleep quality	☐	☐	☐
Stress level	☐	☐	☐
Activity level	☐	☐	☐

Today's goals:
☐ ....
☐ ....
☐ ....

Medications:
☐ ....
☐ ....
☐ ....

Supplements/Nutrition:
☐ ....
☐ ....
☐ ....

Water intake (1 cup = 8 oz)

Coffee I drank today

Juice I drank today

Meditation: from: .... to: .... total minutes: ....

Cardio: from: .... to: .... total calories burn: ....

Exercise: from: .... to: .... total minutes: ....
Type: ....

Daily events
☐ ....   ☐ ....
☐ ....   ☐ ....
☐ ....   ☐ ....

Daily important notes
....
....
....
....
....
....
....

DAILY FOOD LOG

Food	Amount	Cal	Protein	Carbs	Fats	Sugar
Breakfast time:...................						
Lunch time:...................						
Dinner time:...................						
Snacks time:...................						

FOOD TRIGGER TRACKER

Immediately after	After 1 hour	After 3 hours

Symptoms/Pains: ....
....
....
....
....
....
....

DAILY PROGRESS & TRACKER

Date: ....

Day:........... of my journey   Weight: ....

Mo - Tu - We - Th - Fr - Sa - Su

Daily affirmations: ....
....
....

Today mood: 😊 😁 😎 😐 😴 😵 😖

	Low	Medium	High
Energy level	☐	☐	☐
Sleep quality	☐	☐	☐
Stress level	☐	☐	☐
Activity level	☐	☐	☐

Today's goals:
☐ ....
☐ ....
☐ ....

Medications:
☐ ....
☐ ....
☐ ....

Supplements/Nutrition:
☐ ....
☐ ....
☐ ....

Water intake (1 cup = 8 oz)

Coffee I drank today

Juice I drank today

Meditation: from: .... to: .... total minutes: ....

Cardio: from: .... to: .... total calories burn: ....

Exercise: from: .... to: .... total minutes: ....
Type: ....

Daily events
☐ ....   ☐ ....
☐ ....   ☐ ....
☐ ....   ☐ ....

Daily important notes
....
....
....
....
....
....
....

DAILY FOOD LOG

Food	Amount	Cal	Protein	Carbs	Fats	Sugar
Breakfast time:.................						
Lunch time:.................						
Dinner time:.................						
Snacks time:...................						

FOOD TRIGGER TRACKER

Immediately after	After 1 hour	After 3 hours

Symptoms/Pains: ....
....
....
....
....
....
....
....

DAILY PROGRESS & TRACKER

Date: ....

Day: .... of my journey   Weight: ....   Mo - Tu - We - Th - Fr - Sa - Su

Daily affirmations: ....
....
....

Today mood: 😊 😄 😎 🙂 😴 😵 😣

	Low	Medium	High
Energy level	☐	☐	☐
Sleep quality	☐	☐	☐
Stress level	☐	☐	☐
Activity level	☐	☐	☐

Today's goals:
- ☐ ....
- ☐ ....
- ☐ ....

Water intake (1 cup = 8 oz)

Medications:
- ☐ ....
- ☐ ....
- ☐ ....

Coffee I drank today

Supplements/Nutrition:
- ☐ ....
- ☐ ....
- ☐ ....

Juice I drank today

Meditation: from: .... to: .... total minutes: ....

Cardio: from: .... to: .... total calories burn: ....

Exercise: from: .... to: .... total minutes: ....
Type: ....

Daily events
- ☐ ....
- ☐ ....
- ☐ ....
- ☐ ....
- ☐ ....
- ☐ ....

Daily important notes
....
....
....
....
....
....
....
....

DAILY FOOD LOG

Food	Amount	Cal	Protein	Carbs	Fats	Sugar
Breakfast time:...................						
Lunch time:...................						
Dinner time:...................						
Snacks time:						

FOOD TRIGGER TRACKER

Immediately after	After 1 hour	After 3 hours

Symptoms/Pains: ....
....
....
....
....
....
....

DAILY PROGRESS & TRACKER

Date: ....

Day:.......... of my journey   Weight: ....   Mo - Tu - We - Th - Fr - Sa - Su

Daily affirmations: ....
....
....

Today mood: 😊 😄 😎 🙂 😴 😵 😠

	Low	Medium	High
Energy level	☐	☐	☐
Sleep quality	☐	☐	☐
Stress level	☐	☐	☐
Activity level	☐	☐	☐

Today's goals:
☐ ....
☐ ....
☐ ....

Medications:
☐ ....
☐ ....
☐ ....

Supplements/Nutrition:
☐ ....
☐ ....
☐ ....

Water intake (1 cup = 8 oz)

Coffee I drank today

Juice I drank today

Meditation: from: .... to: .... total minutes: ....

Cardio: from: .... to: .... total calories burn:.........................

Exercise: from: .... to: .... total minutes: ....
Type: ....

Daily events
☐ ....   ☐ ....
☐ ....   ☐ ....
☐ ....   ☐ ....

Daily important notes
....
....
....
....
....
....
....

DAILY FOOD LOG

Food	Amount	Cal	Protein	Carbs	Fats	Sugar
Breakfast time:...................						
Lunch time:...................						
Dinner time:...................						
Snacks time:...................						

FOOD TRIGGER TRACKER

Immediately after	After 1 hour	After 3 hours

Symptoms/Pains: ....

....

....

....

....

....

DAILY PROGRESS & TRACKER

Date: ....

Day: .... of my journey   Weight: ....

Mo - Tu - We - Th - Fr - Sa - Su

	Low	Medium	High
Energy level	☐	☐	☐
Sleep quality	☐	☐	☐
Stress level	☐	☐	☐
Activity level	☐	☐	☐

Daily affirmations: ....
....
....

Today mood: 😊 😁 😎 😐 😴 🤪 😖

Today's goals:
☐ ....
☐ ....
☐ ....

Medications:
☐ ....
☐ ....
☐ ....

Supplements/Nutrition:
☐ ....
☐ ....
☐ ....

Water intake (1 cup = 8 oz)

Coffee I drank today

Juice I drank today

Meditation: from: .... to: .... total minutes: ....

Cardio: from: .... to: .... total calories burn: ....

Exercise: from: .... to: .... total minutes: ....
Type: ....

Daily events
☐ ....   ☐ ....
☐ ....   ☐ ....
☐ ....   ☐ ....

Daily important notes
....
....
....
....
....
....
....

DAILY FOOD LOG

Food	Amount	Cal	Protein	Carbs	Fats	Sugar
🍳 Breakfast time:..................						
🌐 Lunch time:..................						
🍳 Dinner time:..................						
🍿 Snacks time:..................						

FOOD TRIGGER TRACKER

Immediately after	After 1 hour	After 3 hours

Symptoms/Pains: ....
....
....
....
....
....
....

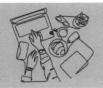

WEEKLY ACTIVITY PLANNER

WEEK OF: ....

WEEKLY CHALLENGES AND GOALS

- [ ] ....
- [ ] ....
- [ ] ....
- [ ] ....
- [ ] ....
- [ ] ....
- [ ] ....
- [ ] ....
- [ ] ....
- [ ] ....
- [ ] ....
- [ ] ....
- [ ] ....
- [ ] ....
- [ ] ....
- [ ] ....
- [ ] ....
- [ ] ....
- [ ] ....
- [ ] ....
- [ ] ....

WEEKLY TO-DO LISTS

- [ ] ....
- [ ] ....
- [ ] ....
- [ ] ....
- [ ] ....
- [ ] ....
- [ ] ....
- [ ] ....
- [ ] ....
- [ ] ....
- [ ] ....
- [ ] ....

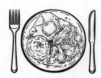

WEEKLY MEAL PLANNER

WEEK OF: ....

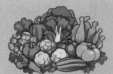

	BREAKFAST	SNACK	LUNCH	DINNER
MON				
TUE				
WED				
THU				
FRI				
SAT				
SUN				

DAILY PROGRESS & TRACKER

Date: ....

Day: .... of my journey   Weight: ....   Mo - Tu - We - Th - Fr - Sa - Su

Daily affirmations: ....
....
....

	Low	Medium	High
Energy level	☐	☐	☐
Sleep quality	☐	☐	☐
Stress level	☐	☐	☐
Activity level	☐	☐	☐

Today mood: 😊 😊 😎 🙂 😴 😵 😣

Today's goals:
- ☐ ....
- ☐ ....
- ☐ ....

Medications:
- ☐ ....
- ☐ ....
- ☐ ....

Supplements/Nutrition:
- ☐ ....
- ☐ ....
- ☐ ....

Water intake (1 cup = 8 oz)

Coffee I drank today

Juice I drank today

Meditation: from: .... to: .... total minutes: ....

Cardio: from: .... to: .... total calories burn: ....

Exercise: from: .... to: .... total minutes: ....
Type: ....

Daily events
- ☐ ....   ☐ ....
- ☐ ....   ☐ ....
- ☐ ....   ☐ ....

Daily important notes
....
....
....
....
....
....
....

DAILY FOOD LOG

Food	Amount	Cal	Protein	Carbs	Fats	Sugar
Breakfast time:...................						
Lunch time:..................						
Dinner time:..................						
Snacks time:						

FOOD TRIGGER TRACKER

Immediately after	After 1 hour	After 3 hours

Symptoms/Pains: ....
....
....
....
....
....
....

DAILY PROGRESS & TRACKER

Date: ....

Day:.......... of my journey   Weight: ....

Mo - Tu - We - Th - Fr - Sa - Su

Daily affirmations: ....
....
....

	Low	Medium	High
Energy level	☐	☐	☐
Sleep quality	☐	☐	☐
Stress level	☐	☐	☐
Activity level	☐	☐	☐

Today mood: 😊 😃 😎 🙂 😴 😵 😠

Today's goals:
☐ ....
☐ ....
☐ ....

Water intake (1 cup = 8 oz)

Medications:
☐ ....
☐ ....
☐ ....

Coffee I drank today

Supplements/Nutrition:
☐ ....
☐ ....
☐ ....

Juice I drank today

Meditation: from: .... to: .... total minutes: ....

Cardio: from: .... to: .... total calories burn: ....

Exercise: from: .... to: .... total minutes: ....
Type: ....

Daily events
☐ ....   ☐ ....
☐ ....   ☐ ....
☐ ....   ☐ ....

Daily important notes
....
....
....
....
....
....
....

DAILY FOOD LOG

Food	Amount	Cal	Protein	Carbs	Fats	Sugar
🍳 Breakfast time:.................						
🌍 Lunch time:.................						
🍽 Dinner time:.................						
🍿 Snacks time:.................						

FOOD TRIGGER TRACKER

Immediately after	After 1 hour	After 3 hours

Symptoms/Pains: ....
....
....
....
....
....
....

DAILY PROGRESS & TRACKER

Date: ....

Day:........... of my journey   Weight: ....   Mo - Tu - We - Th - Fr - Sa - Su

Daily affirmations: ....
....
....

	Low	Medium	High
Energy level	☐	☐	☐
Sleep quality	☐	☐	☐
Stress level	☐	☐	☐
Activity level	☐	☐	☐

Today mood: 😀 😊 😎 🙂 😴 🤢 😖

Today's goals:
- ☐ ....
- ☐ ....
- ☐ ....

Water intake (1 cup = 8 oz)

Medications:
- ☐ ....
- ☐ ....
- ☐ ....

Coffee I drank today

Supplements/Nutrition:
- ☐ ....
- ☐ ....
- ☐ ....

Juice I drank today

Meditation: from: .... to: .... total minutes: ....

Cardio: from: .... to: .... total calories burn: ....

Exercise: from: .... to: .... total minutes: ....
Type: ....

Daily events
- ☐ ....
- ☐ ....
- ☐ ....
- ☐ ....
- ☐ ....
- ☐ ....

Daily important notes
....
....
....
....
....
....
....

DAILY FOOD LOG

Food	Amount	Cal	Protein	Carbs	Fats	Sugar
Breakfast time:..................						
Lunch time:..................						
Dinner time:..................						
Snacks time:						

FOOD TRIGGER TRACKER

Immediately after	After 1 hour	After 3 hours

Symptoms/Pains: ....
....
....
....
....
....
....

DAILY PROGRESS & TRACKER

Date: ....

Day: .... of my journey   Weight: ....   Mo - Tu - We - Th - Fr - Sa - Su

Daily affirmations: ....
....
....

Today mood: 😊 😁 😎 😐 😴 🤪 😵

	Low	Medium	High
Energy level	☐	☐	☐
Sleep quality	☐	☐	☐
Stress level	☐	☐	☐
Activity level	☐	☐	☐

Today's goals:
☐ ....
☐ ....
☐ ....

Medications:
☐ ....
☐ ....
☐ ....

Supplements/Nutrition:
☐ ....
☐ ....
☐ ....

Water intake (1 cup = 8 oz)

Coffee I drank today

Juice I drank today

Meditation: from: .... to: .... total minutes: ....

Cardio: from: .... to: .... total calories burn: ....

Exercise: from: .... to: .... total minutes: ....
Type: ....

Daily events
☐ ....   ☐ ....
☐ ....   ☐ ....
☐ ....   ☐ ....

Daily important notes
....
....
....
....
....
....
....

DAILY FOOD LOG

Food	Amount	Cal	Protein	Carbs	Fats	Sugar
Breakfast time:...................						
Lunch time:...................						
Dinner time:...................						
Snacks time:...................						

FOOD TRIGGER TRACKER

Immediately after	After 1 hour	After 3 hours

Symptoms/Pains: ....
....
....
....
....
....
....

DAILY PROGRESS & TRACKER

Date: ....

Day: .... of my journey   Weight: ....

Mo - Tu - We - Th - Fr - Sa - Su

Daily affirmations: ....
....
....

Today mood: 😊 😄 😎 😐 😴 😵 😖

	Low	Medium	High
Energy level	☐	☐	☐
Sleep quality	☐	☐	☐
Stress level	☐	☐	☐
Activity level	☐	☐	☐

Today's goals:
- ☐ ....
- ☐ ....
- ☐ ....

Medications:
- ☐ ....
- ☐ ....
- ☐ ....

Supplements/Nutrition:
- ☐ ....
- ☐ ....
- ☐ ....

Water intake (1 cup = 8 oz)

Coffee I drank today

Juice I drank today

Meditation: from: .... to: .... total minutes: ....

Cardio: from: .... to: .... total calories burn: ....

Exercise: from: .... to: .... total minutes: ....
Type: ....

Daily events
- ☐ ....
- ☐ ....
- ☐ ....
- ☐ ....
- ☐ ....
- ☐ ....

Daily important notes
....
....
....
....
....
....
....

DAILY FOOD LOG

Food	Amount	Cal	Protein	Carbs	Fats	Sugar
Breakfast time:.................						
Lunch time:.................						
Dinner time:.................						
Snacks time:.................						

FOOD TRIGGER TRACKER

Immediately after	After 1 hour	After 3 hours

Symptoms/Pains: ....
....
....
....
....
....
....

DAILY PROGRESS & TRACKER

Date: ....

Day:.......... of my journey   Weight: ....   Mo - Tu - We - Th - Fr - Sa - Su

Daily affirmations: ....
....
....

Today mood: 😊 😄 😎 🙂 😴 😵 😖

	Low	Medium	High
Energy level	☐	☐	☐
Sleep quality	☐	☐	☐
Stress level	☐	☐	☐
Activity level	☐	☐	☐

Today's goals:
☐ ....
☐ ....
☐ ....

Water intake (1 cup = 8 oz)

Medications:
☐ ....
☐ ....
☐ ....

Coffee I drank today

Supplements/Nutrition:
☐ ....
☐ ....
☐ ....

Juice I drank today

Meditation: from: .... to: .... total minutes: ....

Cardio: from: .... to: .... total calories burn:........................

Exercise: from: .... to: .... total minutes: ....
Type: ....

Daily events
☐ ....   ☐ ....
☐ ....   ☐ ....
☐ ....   ☐ ....

Daily important notes
....
....
....
....
....
....
....
....

DAILY FOOD LOG

Food	Amount	Cal	Protein	Carbs	Fats	Sugar
Breakfast time:..................						
Lunch time:..................						
Dinner time:..................						
Snacks time:..................						

FOOD TRIGGER TRACKER

Immediately after	After 1 hour	After 3 hours

Symptoms/Pains: ....
....
....
....
....
....
....

DAILY PROGRESS & TRACKER

Date: ....

Day:........... of my journey   Weight: ....   Mo - Tu - We - Th - Fr - Sa - Su

Daily affirmations: ....
....
....

	Low	Medium	High
Energy level	☐	☐	☐
Sleep quality	☐	☐	☐
Stress level	☐	☐	☐
Activity level	☐	☐	☐

Today mood: 😄 😊 😎 🙂 😴 😵 😖

Today's goals:
☐ ....
☐ ....
☐ ....

Medications:
☐ ....
☐ ....
☐ ....

Supplements/Nutrition:
☐ ....
☐ ....
☐ ....

Water intake (1 cup = 8 oz)

Coffee I drank today

Juice I drank today

Meditation: from: .... to: .... total minutes: ....

Cardio: from: .... to: .... total calories burn: ....

Exercise: from: .... to: .... total minutes: ....
Type: ....

Daily events
☐ ....   ☐ ....
☐ ....   ☐ ....
☐ ....   ☐ ....

Daily important notes
....
....
....
....
....
....
....
....

DAILY FOOD LOG

Food	Amount	Cal	Protein	Carbs	Fats	Sugar
Breakfast time:..................						
Lunch time:..................						
Dinner time:..................						
Snacks time:..................						

FOOD TRIGGER TRACKER

Immediately after	After 1 hour	After 3 hours

Symptoms/Pains: ....
....
....
....
....
....
....
....

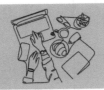

WEEKLY ACTIVITY PLANNER

WEEK OF: ....

WEEKLY CHALLENGES AND GOALS

- ☐ ....
- ☐ ....
- ☐ ....
- ☐ ....
- ☐ ....
- ☐ ....
- ☐ ....
- ☐ ....
- ☐ ....
- ☐ ....
- ☐ ....
- ☐ ....
- ☐ ....
- ☐ ....
- ☐ ....
- ☐ ....
- ☐ ....
- ☐ ....
- ☐ ....
- ☐ ....
- ☐ ....
- ☐ ....

WEEKLY TO-DO LISTS

☐	☐ ....
☐	☐ ....
☐	☐ ....
☐	☐ ....
☐	☐ ....
☐	☐ ....
☐	☐ ....
☐	☐ ....
☐	☐ ....
☐	☐ ....
☐	☐ ....

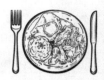

WEEKLY MEAL PLANNER

WEEK OF: ....

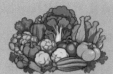

	BREAKFAST	SNACK	LUNCH	DINNER
MON				
TUE				
WED				
THU				
FRI				
SAT				
SUN				

DAILY PROGRESS & TRACKER

Date: ....

Day:.......... of my journey   Weight: ....   Mo - Tu - We - Th - Fr - Sa - Su

Daily affirmations: ....
....
....

Today mood: 😊 😄 😎 🙂 😴 😵 😖

	Low	Medium	High
Energy level	☐	☐	☐
Sleep quality	☐	☐	☐
Stress level	☐	☐	☐
Activity level	☐	☐	☐

Today's goals:
- ☐ ....
- ☐ ....
- ☐ ....

Medications:
- ☐ ....
- ☐ ....
- ☐ ....

Supplements/Nutrition:
- ☐ ....
- ☐ ....
- ☐ ....

Water intake (1 cup = 8 oz)

Coffee I drank today

Juice I drank today

Meditation: from: .... to: .... total minutes: ....

Cardio: from: .... to: .... total calories burn: ....

Exercise: from: .... to: .... total minutes: ....
Type: ....

Daily events
- ☐ ....
- ☐ ....
- ☐ ....
- ☐ ....
- ☐ ....
- ☐ ....

Daily important notes
....
....
....
....
....
....
....

DAILY FOOD LOG

Food	Amount	Cal	Protein	Carbs	Fats	Sugar
Breakfast time:................						
Lunch time:................						
Dinner time:...............						
Snacks time:................						

FOOD TRIGGER TRACKER

Immediately after	After 1 hour	After 3 hours

Symptoms/Pains: ....
....
....
....
....
....
....

DAILY PROGRESS & TRACKER

Date: ....

Day: .... of my journey   Weight: ....   Mo - Tu - We - Th - Fr - Sa - Su

Daily affirmations: ....
....
....

	Low	Medium	High
Energy level	☐	☐	☐
Sleep quality	☐	☐	☐
Stress level	☐	☐	☐
Activity level	☐	☐	☐

Today mood: 😊 😄 😎 🙂 😌 😵 😖

Today's goals:
- ☐ ....
- ☐ ....
- ☐ ....

Water intake (1 cup = 8 oz)

Medications:
- ☐ ....
- ☐ ....
- ☐ ....

Coffee I drank today

Supplements/Nutrition:
- ☐ ....
- ☐ ....
- ☐ ....

Juice I drank today

Meditation: from: .... to: .... total minutes: ....

Cardio: from: .... to: .... total calories burn: ....

Exercise: from: .... to: .... total minutes: ....
Type: ....

Daily events
- ☐ .... ☐ ....
- ☐ .... ☐ ....
- ☐ .... ☐ ....

Daily important notes
....
....
....
....
....
....
....
....

DAILY FOOD LOG

Food	Amount	Cal	Protein	Carbs	Fats	Sugar
Breakfast time:................						
Lunch time:................						
Dinner time:................						
Snacks time:................						

FOOD TRIGGER TRACKER

Immediately after	After 1 hour	After 3 hours

Symptoms/Pains: ....

....

....

....

....

....

....

DAILY PROGRESS & TRACKER

Date: ....

Day:........... of my journey   Weight: ....

Mo - Tu - We - Th - Fr - Sa - Su

Daily affirmations: ....
....
....

Today mood: 😊 😄 😎 😐 😴 😵 😣

	Low	Medium	High
Energy level	☐	☐	☐
Sleep quality	☐	☐	☐
Stress level	☐	☐	☐
Activity level	☐	☐	☐

Today's goals:
☐ ....
☐ ....
☐ ....

Medications:
☐ ....
☐ ....
☐ ....

Supplements/Nutrition:
☐ ....
☐ ....
☐ ....

Water intake (1 cup = 8 oz)

Coffee I drank today

Juice I drank today

Meditation: from: .... to: .... total minutes: ....

Cardio: from: .... to: .... total calories burn: ....

Exercise: from: .... to: .... total minutes: ....
Type: ....

Daily events
☐ ....   ☐ ....
☐ ....   ☐ ....
☐ ....   ☐ ....

Daily important notes
....
....
....
....
....
....
....

DAILY FOOD LOG

Food	Amount	Cal	Protein	Carbs	Fats	Sugar
🍳 Breakfast time:...............						
🌍 Lunch time:...............						
🍽 Dinner time:...............						
🍿 Snacks time:...............						

FOOD TRIGGER TRACKER

Immediately after	After 1 hour	After 3 hours

Symptoms/Pains: ....
....
....
....
....
....
....

DAILY PROGRESS & TRACKER

Date: ....

Day:............ of my journey   Weight: ....

Mo - Tu - We - Th - Fr - Sa - Su

Daily affirmations: ....
....
....

Today mood: 😊 😁 😎 😐 😳 😵 😖

	Low	Medium	High
Energy level	☐	☐	☐
Sleep quality	☐	☐	☐
Stress level	☐	☐	☐
Activity level	☐	☐	☐

Today's goals:
☐ ....
☐ ....
☐ ....

Medications:
☐ ....
☐ ....
☐ ....

Supplements/Nutrition:
☐ ....
☐ ....
☐ ....

Water intake (1 cup = 8 oz)

Coffee I drank today

Juice I drank today

Meditation: from: .... to: .... total minutes: ....

Cardio: from: .... to: .... total calories burn: ....

Exercise: from: .... to: .... total minutes: ....
Type: ....

Daily events
☐ ....   ☐ ....
☐ ....   ☐ ....
☐ ....   ☐ ....

Daily important notes
....
....
....
....
....
....
....

DAILY FOOD LOG

Food	Amount	Cal	Protein	Carbs	Fats	Sugar
Breakfast time:...................						
Lunch time:...................						
Dinner time:...................						
Snacks time:...................						

FOOD TRIGGER TRACKER

Immediately after	After 1 hour	After 3 hours

Symptoms/Pains: ....
....
....
....
....
....
....

DAILY PROGRESS & TRACKER

Date: ....

Day: .... of my journey   Weight: ....

Mo - Tu - We - Th - Fr - Sa - Su

Daily affirmations: ....
....
....

Today mood: 😊 😄 😎 🙂 😴 😵 😣

	Low	Medium	High
Energy level	☐	☐	☐
Sleep quality	☐	☐	☐
Stress level	☐	☐	☐
Activity level	☐	☐	☐

Today's goals:
☐ ....
☐ ....
☐ ....

Medications:
☐ ....
☐ ....
☐ ....

Supplements/Nutrition:
☐ ....
☐ ....
☐ ....

Water intake (1 cup = 8 oz)

Coffee I drank today

Juice I drank today

Meditation: from: .... to: .... total minutes: ....

Cardio: from: .... to: .... total calories burn: ....

Exercise: from: .... to: .... total minutes: ....
Type: ....

Daily events
☐ ....   ☐ ....
☐ ....   ☐ ....
☐ ....   ☐ ....

Daily important notes
....
....
....
....
....
....
....

DAILY FOOD LOG

Food	Amount	Cal	Protein	Carbs	Fats	Sugar
Breakfast time:................						
Lunch time:................						
Dinner time:................						
Snacks time:................						

FOOD TRIGGER TRACKER

Immediately after	After 1 hour	After 3 hours

Symptoms/Pains: ....

....

....

....

....

....

....

DAILY PROGRESS & TRACKER

Date: ....

Day:.......... of my journey   Weight: ....

Mo - Tu - We - Th - Fr - Sa - Su

Daily affirmations: ....
....
....

Today mood: 😊 😄 😎 😐 😴 😵 😖

	Low	Medium	High
Energy level	☐	☐	☐
Sleep quality	☐	☐	☐
Stress level	☐	☐	☐
Activity level	☐	☐	☐

Today's goals:
- ☐ ....
- ☐ ....
- ☐ ....

Medications:
- ☐ ....
- ☐ ....
- ☐ ....

Supplements/Nutrition:
- ☐ ....
- ☐ ....
- ☐ ....

Water intake (1 cup = 8 oz)

Coffee I drank today

Juice I drank today

Meditation: from: .... to: .... total minutes: ....

Cardio: from: .... to: .... total calories burn: ....

Exercise: from: .... to: .... total minutes: ....
Type: ....

Daily events
- ☐ ....
- ☐ ....
- ☐ ....
- ☐ ....
- ☐ ....
- ☐ ....

Daily important notes
....
....
....
....
....
....
....

DAILY FOOD LOG

Food	Amount	Cal	Protein	Carbs	Fats	Sugar
🍳 Breakfast time:...................						
🌐 Lunch time:...................						
🍳 Dinner time:...................						
🍿 Snacks time:...................						

FOOD TRIGGER TRACKER

Immediately after	After 1 hour	After 3 hours

Symptoms/Pains: ....
....
....
....
....
....
....

DAILY PROGRESS & TRACKER

Date: ....

Day:........... of my journey   Weight: ....

Mo - Tu - We - Th - Fr - Sa - Su

	Low	Medium	High
Energy level	☐	☐	☐
Sleep quality	☐	☐	☐
Stress level	☐	☐	☐
Activity level	☐	☐	☐

Daily affirmations: ....
....
....

Today mood: ☺ ☺ 😎 ☺ 😴 😵 😖

Today's goals:

☐ ....
☐ ....
☐ ....

Medications:

☐ ....
☐ ....
☐ ....

Supplements/Nutrition:

☐ ....
☐ ....
☐ ....

Water intake (1 cup = 8 oz)

Coffee I drank today

Juice I drank today

Meditation: from: .... to: .... total minutes: ....

Cardio: from: .... to: .... total calories burn:........................

Exercise: from: .... to: ....total minutes: ....
Type: ....

Daily events

☐ ....   ☐ ....
☐ ....   ☐ ....
☐ ....   ☐ ....

Daily important notes

....
....
....
....
....
....
....

DAILY FOOD LOG

Food	Amount	Cal	Protein	Carbs	Fats	Sugar
🍳 Breakfast time:...................						
🌐 Lunch time:						
🍳 Dinner time:................						
🍿 Snacks time:						

FOOD TRIGGER TRACKER

Immediately after	After 1 hour	After 3 hours

Symptoms/Pains: ....
....
....
....
....
....
....

Write a short story about your Bariatric Surgery journey from start to finish. How did you struggle, what was the hardest thing to achieve, and what motivated you the most to move forward until you succeed today?

....
....
....
....
....
....
....
....
....
....
....
....
....
....
....
....
....
....
....
....
....
....
....
....
....
....
....
....
....
....
....
....
....
....
....

Made in United States
Troutdale, OR
04/24/2024

19411158R00077